HearthMath Affinity 1

Dragana Dj. Jeremic

dragana@relax8.space

https://relax8.space

Independent Publishing

Limits of Liability and Disclaimer of Warranty

The author and publisher shall not be liable for your misuse of this material. This book is strictly for informational and educational purposes.

Warning – Disclaimer

The purpose of this book is to educate and entertain. The author and/or publisher do not guarantee that anyone following these techniques, suggestions, tips, ideas, or strategies will become successful. The author and/or publisher shall have neither liability nor responsibility to anyone with respect to any loss or damage caused, or alleged to be caused, directly or indirectly by the information contained in this book.

"True belonging doesn't require you to change who you are; it requires you to be who you are."

~ Brené Brown

COVER PHOTO BY DRAGANA DJ. JEREMIC

The University Library Svetozar Markovic in Belgrade was built partially by Dale Carnegie's donation. He was one of the richest men in the world (1835 -1919) who dedicated up to 90 percent of his wealth to philanthropy. In fact, 100.000 USD were granted to Serbian Government and that amounts to approximately one third of the cost of the library in total. One of the influential individuals involved in the project was Mihajlo Pupin (1854–1935), who was a professor of physics at the Columbia University.

The library is still one of the favourite places for young people as well as lifelong learners. I find it very user friendly for it is open from 8 a.m. to 8 p.m. on workdays and from 8 a.m. to 2 p.m. on Saturdays.

Key words: University Library in Belgrade; Serbia; Carnegie Libraries; Gable or Pediment; Svetozar Markovic

https://en.wikipedia.org/wiki/Belgrade_University_Library

https://www.britannica.com/technology/gable

http://www.unilib.rs/

Dragana Dj. Jeremic used to study occasionally In the Carnegie
Library in Belgrade. This was beneficial time for she has managed
to acquire several degrees. Firstly, she graduated LLB degree (four
years) at Faculty of Laws, University of Belgrade, Republic of
Serbia, the degree number is #40809, dated 22.IV 1994,
She also achieved magister degree (three years) at the same Faculty,
#834, dated 26.12.1997 which was published on the page 616, #9
of the Annals of the Faculty of Law in Belgrade, Year XLV, no. 4-
6, July-December 1997, pp. 321-640/UDC 34/35, YU-ISSN 0003-
2565. Impressive, the Annalies has been published since 1906.
https://anali.rs/?lang=en

Next, Dragana Dj. Jeremic graduated Psychology at Faculty of
Communication and Media Studies, Singidunum University,
Belgrade, Republic of Serbia, #530, dated 16.05.2014 and Master's
Degree in Psychology, # I 151/14, dated 27.06.2015.

Finally, Dragana also holds license for graduated jurists #130-152-
02-1279/2015-06 dated 23.12.2015 issued by the Ministry of Public
Administration and Local Self-Government, Republic of Serbia
https://mduls.gov.rs/en/home/ as well as the license issued by the
Ministry of Health of the Republic of Serbia for Graduated
Psychologists, #152-02-1104/2015-04 dated 01.09.2015
https://www.zdravlje.gov.rs/.

.

Gift to my readers: Mini Workbook PDF

Habitual emotions tend to be long-standing. Moreover, sometimes they are hidden, so it might be advantageous to follow throw on the process which contains several steps. As a result, we are about to acknowledge what domains are critical as well as specific factors which often trigger emotional reaction. Whether you choose to consider that in a form of peaceful contemplation or conversations with friends, the final step is practicing one HeartMath technique of your choice.

Here is the link for a gift companion to Dragana's book *HeartMath Affinity 1*.

https://relax8.space/gift-affinity-1/

Please keep the link private. You may wish to review her Amazon author page:

https://amazon.com/author/draganajoy

I am glad we could create the online relationship. You may send me an email to

dragana@relax8.space

Review request

I appreciate that we spent time together engaging with "HeartMath Affinity 1". If you found this book helpful, I would be grateful for your review.

Welcome to my Amazon author page

https://amazon.com/author/draganajoy

Find the title "HeartMath Affinity 1", scroll down and click WRITE A CUSTOMER REVIEW button. Every vote is important. You may opt for stars only.

Alternatively, another choice is writing one or several sentences to post the review.

Leaving a rating for Dragana's books on will help other people find this book. You'll also support an independent author Dragana by posting your review.

About the Author

Dragana Dj. Jeremic is a master psychologist, master jurist, photographer and English instructor among other hats she is keen on wearing as a life-long learner as well as spiritual seeker.

She has become the Certified HeartMath Practitioner in 2024, after exploring HearhMath technics for several years. https://certified.heartmath.com/user/dragana-jeremic/

CONTENTS

1) INTRODUCTION

Some people who would like to be regarded as my potential clients ask me about certain aspects of *the HeartMath(r) Resiliency* course I am certified for. Often these individuals claim the did not suffer from trauma but have certain everday challenges which may have lasted for a long time. Although they reject any connection to a traumatic experience, those people request help for persistently failing at specific goals. Moreover, they used to become irritated at any attempt to soften the expression "failure" they use harshly. For instance, the idea that between failure and success the crucial difference is whether a person gives up or not, meaning keep on working on your aim or tweak it a little and you might succeed, too.

In essence, that type of my potential client is not very flexible. I assume there are two paths for us to proceed if both sides choose to do so. On one hand, we may disregard trauma and focus on specific aspects which might have shown up in their lives as obstacles to achieving that goal. Due to the fact that the are familiar with the Law of Attraction, they are willing to talk using the LoA expressions which is acceptable to me. On the other hand, I may try to explain fundamental ideas on traumatic experience in order to check whether these frustrating factors in their lives mirror trauma or not.

Obviously, clients who did not endure any trauma might use the same approach. Having studied the regular Law of Attraction literature, they are unaccustomed to this HeartMath approach hence it could be even more compelling to them.

2) WHAT IS TRAUMA?

Clients who tend to reject any chance of suffering from trauma do not talk about two types of traumas: one is with the capital 'T' and the other is with the lower-case 't'. The former refers to stressors such as natural disasters, wars and other obviously detrimental events that may have happened to them. It is vital to notice not only that there is another type of trauma, but also that in undesirable circumstances, not everyone reacts alike. That is, the reaction to stress is subjective, "Stress is a state of burdened response to stressors, resulted in deterioration and dysfunction" (Selye, 1956). Meaning, having felt these events were so dangerous that they could have died or been physically hurt, they end up feeling afraid, helpless or terrified. For example, a number of people become victims of those adverse events, while others recover relatively fast and without displaying any long-lasting consequences.

The lower-case trauma stands for "little events" which might have happened to us on many occasions. Even though some people have treated those as natural part of life, the effect may be adverse and long-standing. "Multiple exposures to traumatic event can greatly affect the intensity of not only the psychological symptoms but also the physical symptoms" (Andrea et al., 2011, p.379). If clients were severely affected by so called "regular everyday circumstances", we may talk about trauma. Whereas groups of adults disregarded that option, others were willing to work with me on establishing the intensity of feasible trauma.

In this book, we deal with people who deny they have suffered from trauma but are willing to work on their long-term blocks to achieve chosen goals as well as those who prefer HeartMath perspective regardless of trauma.

3) What is Your Habitual Emotion?

Most of us have a familiar emotion that we tend to feel most of the time. In terms of the Low of Attraction, that would be our dominant signal. In other words, we contemplate our regular vibration. If that used to be a depleting emotion, it would compete with the specific elevated emotions which have been required for the goal achievement. As a result, we tend to send mixed vibrations. For example, a dominant feeling is fear or anxiety, but we practise enthusiasm three times a day and gratitude regarding our goals. In view of the LoA, that would be sending confusing messages or orders which might undermine our intention.

a) How could we tackle the problem of confusing messages?

In my opinion, it is necessary to transform the dominant emotion which tends to be one of draining emotions such as anger or sadness. It is worth noting that those emotions affect whether we are aware of them or not. "Lower acceptance of emotions was associated with the highest depressive symptoms regardless of suppression or gender" (Flynn, Hollenstein and Mackey, 2010, p. 582). For instance, an individual might express anger openly but suppress sadness.

Whilst emotions that drain our energy are common, we may cultivate regenerating emotions, including excitement and contentment. As a *HeartMath® Certified Practitioner*, I would recommend *Depletion to* Renewal™ *Plan* (2008, 2017, p.1). This is a procedure consisting of six steps covering various elements vital to goal achievement. Additionally, it allows us to display our cognitive intelligence and improve our decision-making. According to Stefanie Veraghen, "These tools enhance your ability to think clearly and navigate daily stressors with ease" (Veraghen, n.d. https://yourhealthandwellbeing.org/event/how-to-go-from-emotional-depletion-to-renewal-2/). Therefore, I believe it is clear why this tool is sometimes called *Emotional Landscape*. Not only it allows us a good overview of emotions, but also may lead to profound effect on our performance and well-being.

b) Two hormones: Cortisol and DHEA

The good news is that if a client applied it properly, that practice could increase his or her level of resiliency. It is related to two hormones called cortisol and DHEA. "Evidently the biochemical interactions between cortisol and DHEA have proven to be of great importance in the determination of declining functions of biological systems" (Ahmed, Quassem, and Kyriacou, 2023, p. 29). In short, depleting emotions are known to increase the level of stress hormone called cortisol which may have a long-lasting effect on our functioning, while renewing emotions are related to "DHEA" which is called a vitality hormone. Therefore, the results of this practice might have not only beneficial effects on our set goals and decision making, but also on our health and vitality.

4) CULTIVATING SELF-COMPASSION

When we engage in negative self-talk it is usually discouraging. Therefore, it is necessary to explore other options, such as taking some time off, remembering our successes and being kind to ourselves. Some people find it irritating or even construct it as a waste of time. Moreover, when challenged with the notion of self-compassions, those individuals may disregard it in various ways, including stating that it is for children only, lack of time is the master in that realm or their friends were talking about it, but it seemed irrelavant.

a) Is it perfect?

Idealization seems to be getting in our way from time to time. I would say because we live in a relative universe, it is natural that we are not perfect. While others could argue there is a potential for perfection in everyone, I think we need to appreciate various levels of reality, or we might disregard some of them. Whereas ideal can be in the absolute realm of existence, our Planet Earth is more related to the relative one. Otherwise, when anything less than optimal shows up, we might end up criticizing ourselves which hinders goal accomplishment.

b) What is Self-Compassion?

To my mind, self-compassion is worth exploring generally, and especially when we are dealing with persistant resistance and so-called failure. According to Kristin Neff, "self-compassion as comprised of six different elements: increased self-kindness, common humanity, and mindfulness as well as reduced self-judgment, isolation, and over-identification" (Neff, 2023, p. 193). First, we need to recognize there is some form of suffering, dissatisfaction or failure as well as that this is a regular part of being a human. In other words, I do not identify with that as a perfect result, event or circumstance because I am able to observe it as just one temporary element in my life. Next, it is not a unique experience that happened only to me for I am in good company of fellow humans who also need to revise and correct their documents or are disappointed again. Finally, we might choose to be kinder not only to others, but also to ourselves.

Even though there are various options when it comes to cultivating self-compassion and self-kindness, I believe that the first step is to recognize its importance. One method is by becoming aware of its effects, "In Study 3, self-compassion moderated negative emotions after receiving ambivalent feedback, particularly for participants who were low in self-esteem" (Leary and al., 2007, p. 887). Following, we need to find a suitable approach to cultivating self-compassion. Nowadays, there are several websites which offer that, so it might be useful to contemplate HeartMath approach not only to compassion, but also how to find the appropriate information and make the beneficial decisions.

c) Heart Lock-In technique

There are some basic HeartMath techniques which encourage self-care such as Heart-Focused Breading and Quick-Coherence as explained online and in my previous book called *Becoming HearMath Practitioner*, sections 2b and 3c, respectively (Jeremic, 2024). In a sense, they are reiterated in steps one and two of this new technique. We may consider self-care as a foundation for self-compassion; it might be useful to inquire our beliefs in that respect. Is it selfish, hedonistic or unproductive to dedicate time, space and money to yourself? By gently practicing these breathing exercises we may open to a different way of thinking and feeling.

Actual steps of the Heart Lock-In technique: Firstly, you are aware of the heart area and you breathe as if the breath is flowing in and out through the heart. It is good to do it slightly slower and deeper that we usually breathe and feel a rhythm of let's say breathing in to the count of five and exhaling for another five seconds. Secondly, you focus on a regenerative feeling such as care, appreciation or compassion towards yourself. Maintain that feeling while repeating the first step for at least one minute. Thirdly, radiate that feeling to any challenge which appeared in your life. Find the balance between observing the problem as it is and sending it renewing feeling.

Impressively, this HeartMath exercise could be performed in many beneficial ways. There are slight tweaks which all might be helpful to you. For instance, we may first introduce the dominant feeling like shame, self-pity or self-judgment and simply accept it. Then do the first two steps with any other renewing feeling, such as gratitude, being proud of accomplishments or courage. In the third step we radiate that feeling to ourselves and naturally move to a higher-level emotion.

d) Self-compassion and Weight management

It is compelling that an overweight person may include compassion techniques as an integral part of this transitional period in his or her life. "The women who gave themselves permission to eat didn't overeat" (Parker-Pope, February 28, 2011 5:26 pm, referring to Adams, Leary, 2007, https://archive.nytimes.com/well.blogs.nytimes.com/2011/02/28/go-easy-on-yourself-a-new-wave-of-research-urges/?partner=rss&emc=rss). Similarly, participants in a study who used diaries in a concrete way focusing on the food and how they were eating as a form of mindfulness, had better results that the other group three months after the study (Mantzios and Willson, 2014, p. 422). It is likely that practising other techniques which promote being aware of what is going on/observing it as one aspect of life, are helpful as opposed to either avoiding the situation or over-identifying with it.

Stopping Emotional Eating is HeartMath book which shows us how to deal with emotional stress and emotional eating. In the first part crucial topics like inner critic, perfectionism as well as sleep, boredom and loneliness are explained in relation to weight regime. It may be surprising that boredom and loneliness are not only included in emotions, but also as indicators of covering up something. If we were willing to use HeartMath tools to discover what that is, it would possibly reveal factors which also trigger overeating. Part two is dedicated to well known Heartmath breathing techniques as well as specific tools including writing exercises, tables and HM technology. Authors Doc Childre and Debora Rozman, PH. D. with Sheva Carr communicate directly to the readers which may be unusual at first. There is no doubt that stress is crucial, which may provoke "weight gain related to elevated stress hormones even in the absence of overeating" (Childre, Rozman, with Carr, 2017, p.13). In essence, learning in what ways to neutralize stressful thoughts and allowing more ease into our lives could be game changers.

5) CONCLUSION

In this book, we have considered the question of people who deny they had to put up with trauma, but want to use HeartMath sessions to overcome barriers to aim fulfillment. First, we discussed two types of traumas, then we focused on our dominant emotions and whether they are in harmony with those required for goal achievement. If not, we may be sending mixed messages, which is detrimental to our intention fulfillment. Therefore, we explore HeartMath tools that might tackle the problem of feeling emotions which are not aligned. Impressively, any individual who is interested in this HeartMath approach might find it beneficial.

Finally, we explored self-compassion or the lack of it. Relevant factors include perfectionism as well as in what ways we understand self-compassion and what it is comprised of. While Heart Lock-In technique and its variations could contribute to enhanced compassion towards self in general, there are specific HeartMath tools in relation to reduction of excess weight.

REFERENCES

Adams, C. E., and Leary, M. R. (2007). Promoting self-compassionate attitudes toward eating among restrictive and guilty eaters. *Journal of Social and Clinical Psychology, 26*(10), 1120–1144. https://doi.org/10.1521/jscp.2007.26.10.1120

Ahmed, T., Quassem, M. and Kyriacou, P. A. (2023). Measuring stress: a review of the current cortisol and dehydroepiandrosterone (DHEA) measurement techniques and considerations for the future of mental health monitoring. *The International Journal on the Biology of Stress, Volume 26, (1).* Pages 29-42. https://www.tandfonline.com/doi/epdf/10.1080/10253890.2022.2164187?needAccess=true

Andrea, W. D., Sharma, R., Zelechoski A. D. and Spinazzola, J. (2011). Physical Health Problems After Single Trauma Exposure: When Stress Takes Root in the Body. *Journal of the American Psychiatric Nurses Association 17(6).* 378-392.

Childre, D., Rozman, D., with Carr, Sh., (2017).
*STOPPING EMOTIONAL EATING: Heartmath(r)
Stress and Weight Management Program.* Boulder
Creek, California: HeartMath(r).

Depletion to Renewal™ Plan. (2008, 2017). Boulder
Creek, California: HeartMath(r).

Felitti, V. J, Anda, A. F., Nordenberg, D., Williamson, D.
F., Spitz, A. M., Edwards, V., Koss, M. P. and
Marks, J. S. (1998). Relationship of Childhood
Abuse and Household Dysfunction to Many of the
Leading causes of Death in Adults. The Adverse
Childhood Experiences (ACE) study. *American
Journal of Preventive medicine. 14(4)*, pages 245-
258.

Flynn, J.J., Hollenstein, T., and Mackey, A. (2010). The
effect of suppressing and not accepting emotions
on depressive symptoms: Is suppression different
for men and women? *Personality and Individual
Differences. 49 (6).* Pages 582-586.
https://doi.org/10.1016/j.paid.2010.05.022

Jeremic, D., (2024). *Becoming HeartMath Practitioner.* Seatle, Washington: Amazon.

Leary, M. R., Tate, E. B., Adams, C. E., Batts Allen, A. and Hancock, J. (2007). Self-compassion and reactions to unpleasant self-relevant events: The implications of treating oneself kindly. *Journal of Personality and Social Psychology, 92*(5), 887–904. https://doi.org/10.1037/0022-3514.92.5.887

Mantzios, M. and Willson, J. C. (2014). Making concrete constructs mindful: a novel approach for developing mindfulness and self-compassion to assist weight loss. *Psychol Health .29(4)*: 422-41. doi: 10.1080/08870446.2013.863883. Epub 2013 Dec 4.

Neff, K. D. (2023). Self-Compassion: Theory, Method, Research, and Intervention. *Annual Review of Psychology 74*: 193–218.

Parker-Pope, T. (February 28, 2011 5:26 pm). *Go Easy on Yourself, a New Wave of Research Urges* https://archive.nytimes.com/well.blogs.nytimes.com/2011/02/28/go-easy-on-yourself-a-new-wave-of-research-urges/?partner=rss&emc=rss).

Selye , H. (1956*). The Stress of Life.* New York City, NY: McGraw-Hill,.

Veraghen, S. (n. d.). *How to Go from Emotional Depletion to Renewal.* Center for Health & Weellbeing. https://yourhealthandwellbeing.org/event/how-to-go-from-emotional-depletion-to-renewal-2/

ALSO, BY DRAGANA DJ. JEREMIC ON AMAZON

Pawsome Friends: A Community Book Project

The book is created by Donna Kozik and 100+ contributing authors. As one of the contributing authors Dragana DJ. Jeremic wrote a short essay and a quote on the pet.

Another community book on gratitude is going to be published soon and Dragana DJ Jeremic wrote her short essay titled Meditation and Action.

Stress, Relaxation and Coloring Books: Peacefulness for Busy People

The stress response should be short and efficient when you are in danger. However, in modern culture people are under stress most of the time. Do you recognize the consequences of long-term stress?

If you practice relaxation techniques daily, you'll probably gain a different mode of functioning. The relaxation response leads to a higher quality of life. Meaning, you might manifest your life priorities and feel better if you are out of the prolonged stress reaction.

Dragana's Five Fantasy Coloring books

Dragana DJ. Jeremic is glad to inform you about her new fantasy coloring system named DETERMINED coloring book.

First, we have several perspectives. Each perspective is a different visual representation of the main theme. Alternatively, we may deal with only one perspective in an easy approach to fantasy coloring books.

Second, Dragana presents each perspective on three levels based on the number and size of the main elements, here cherry blossoms. We may compare it to an establishing shot, American shot and close up in the film industry.

Third, Dragana adds the fantasy elements to each level. There are three versions of each level. We explore white flowers with fantasy pattern environment. Next, we focus on symbol patterns of flowers with natural environment. Finally, we pay attention to mandala pattern flowers with natural environment.

We are going to explore vital ideas of Healing Touch(r) and its numerous tools. As Dragana is in the process of enhancing her knowledge and skills in relation to QT, you will have peer perspective for Dragana believes we learn faster that way. As a certified Quantum Touch Level 1 practitioner and a member of QT Healing Circles as well as QT groups, Dragana will present you with techniques which seem to be fun and powerful, such as Hands on healing, Distant healing, 12 chakras and Toning.

Following, we will explore an alternative view on the Low of Attraction. Having practiced the LoA for some time, you may have found it confusing. Therefore, we are going to consider Richard Gordon's take on this creative subject. He is the founder of the QT modality, and his advice is to create the desired outcomes from the future. If you were like me, meaning creating it as an experience in the past and enjoying the benefits in the present, you could discover valuable tweaks in that respect.

In this book Dragana shares her learning experience prior to acquiring HeartMath Certified Practitioner status in the summer 2024. She has been studying engaging online courses and other materials since 2019 with excellent leaders, such as Deborah Rozman, Howard Martin, Rollin McCraty, Gregg Braden and Jorina Elbers. You might be interested in how Rozman and Braden tweak the same HeartMath exercise.

Following, various details are included, hence you may have a wider perspective on the HeartMath experience. You will also find out in what ways Dragana interacts with clients in 1:1 sessions and group settings.

Finally, she believes that it is important to appreciate both Heart and Brain. When they are in harmony, we are more likely to be healthy, successful and happier in our relationships.

Review request

I appreciate that we spent time together engaging with
"HeathMath Affinity 1". If you found this book helpful, I
would be grateful for your review.
Welcome to my Amazon author page
https://amazon.com/author/draganajoy
Find the title "HeartMath Affinity 1", scroll down and
  click
WRITE A CUSTOMER REVIEW button. Every vote is
  important. You may opt
for stars only. Alternatively, another choice is writing one
  or several sentences to
post the review.
Leaving a rating for Dragana's books on will help other
  people find this book.
You'll also support an independent author Dragana by

  posting your review.

Tryout page

If you would like to try your ideas before working on the desired goals, this page is a good start.

9 798300 707026